Baby Sleep Tra
Days Or L

The Step-By-Step Solution To Teach Your Baby To Stop Crying And Sleep 8-12 Hours Every Night!- EASY AND EFFORTLESSLY

Ally Cooper

Table Of Contents

Chapter 1: How To Begin.. **1**

Chapter 2: Feeding Strategies **7**

Chapter 3: Babies & Sleep **11**

Chapter 4: Feeding Facts **19**

Chapter 5: Your Baby's Day..................................... **30**

Chapter 6: When Baby Cries.................................... **53**

Chapter 7: Colic, Reflux & Inconsolable Babies.. **61**

Chapter 1

HOW TO BEGIN

The home: Nothing will impact a persons life more than the influence parents have on the home environment

The challenge: most couples enter parenthood hoping they will just "know" what to do without putting effort into learning the parenting basics. This goes beyond those Classroom preparations.

For Mom: Physical and Emotional challenges. Before, the protecting and nurturing was taken care of by the in-utero relationship with the baby. All the fine details and baby sounds trigger emotions never previously experienced and she will be overwhelmed by the nurturing, protecting and provisional sensations for her baby

For Dad: Time. Sharing his time with his wife and child. Giving up time with her for time with the child

What about the baby? becomes paramount over any other plans & routines.

One of two false assumptions are usually made: one, that life will not change when the baby arrives, or two, that your peaceful life will descend into a hopeless state of incessant chaos.

Whats Missing?

Most parents begin parenting with high hopes and the best

intentions. They've done research and know a lot of baby facts, but don't understand how the whole picture fits together.

Facts provide a plan, understanding is what provides purpose.

Build a loving home environment:

1. **Your home must be parent-led, NOT child-led:** developmental achievements are too valuable to be left to chance
2. **Falling in love with your baby does not equal providing your baby with a loving home environment** - A healthy home environment starts with Mom & Dad's commitment to each other, from which love is then communicated to the child
3. **I loving home environment does not emerge naturally.** Parents must be intentional in there love for each other. They must also understand the 3 influences that shape every child's destiny:

    1. **Genetic Disposition:** Physical & Intellectual potential
    2. **Temperament:** Dimension of the personality
    3. **The Home Environment created by the Parents:** The first two are out of the parent's control, but the home environment is entirely in control of the parents and is equally as important in development as the other two.

Marriage/Partnership:

No one is born a good husband or wife, they become that way through selflessness, patience & commitment to the happiness and welfare of the other.

You achieve long-term happiness in marriage, you don't find long-term happiness in marriage.

A loving relationship creates a loving home environment which will influence the destiny of the child.

Though your baby cannot yet speak and maturely process all the information in their environment yet, what they observe feeds their developmental psyche.

Observing a healthy relationship provides children with a layer of love & security that cannot be achieved through the direct parent-child relationship - even at an infant stage

Warning: Don't lose sight of the big picture

It is easy to get lost in parenting wonderland: pictures, videos, first words, first steps etc. The baby becomes central to their existence and begins to exclude their relationship as a couple.

The greatest overall influence parents have on their child is not their roles as individual parents, but in their shared role as husband & wife.

When a child observes the friendship & emotional togetherness of the parents, he is naturally more secure because of the confidence in their relationship and the stability of the household. Strong relationships provide a haven of security for children as they mature.

Volatile and bad relationships create a hostile home environment and infuse insecurity into the children. They then search for the relationship between siblings to reflect the lacking stability of the parents relationship

Parents define the meaning of love, security, stability and confidence my the household they create; which is created through their relationship.

Healthy parenting grows from healthy relationships

How do you keep your relationship alive and well to maximize your parenting influence?

1. **Continue Living.** Life does not stop when the baby arrives. It may slow down for the first few weeks, but it is important to keep on living
2. **Don't stop Dating.** Your weekly date night doesn't stop when the baby arrives, you are still a couple and need to keep doing what made your relationship special
3. Continue what you love. Did you have a tradition or special activity you enjoyed before the baby arrived? Plan it into your schedule. They are what make your relationship special, and need to be kept special.
4. **Talk Time.** Spend at least 15 un-interrupted min 4-5 days/week sitting together with your spouse discussing the days events and beyond. Let your child play while mom and dad are having their time together. This keeps a visual demonstration of your love for each other and the value you both have on your relationship with each other at the forefront of your parenting which the child intuitively understands, appreciates and finds security in.
5. **Know what to expect before the baby arrives.** Delegate duties of seemingly menial tasks before hand so that you can minimize stress in the first few weeks - especially if you are expecting your first child.

Home

- Wash Laundry
- fold laundry
- put away laundry
- ironing
- dry cleaning
- groceries
- putting away Groceries
- Preparing Meals
- Breakfast
- Lunch
- Dinner
- Wash Dishes
- Load Dishwasher
- Home Care
- Clean Bathroom
- Vacuum
- Dust
- Make Bed
- Change Sheets
- Water Plants
- Take out Trash/Recycling
- Pet Feeding
- Walking Dog/ Pet Clean Up
- Yard Work
- Getting the Mail
- Paying Bills
- Banking
- Vehicle Maintenance/Service
- etc. and others

Baby-Care

- Feed Baby (If Bottle Fed)
- Diaper Changes
- Get Baby For Night Feeding
- Night Feeding (If Bottle Fed)
- Baby Bathing
- Comforting Fussy Baby
- Care of Other Children
- etc. and others

Single Parents:

Single parents face double duty with the care and responsibility of raising a child.

You love your baby with the same passion as any couple, and desire to give your baby the best chance in life. It is our privilege to help all parents maximize their emotional & intellectual resources, regardless of marital status or orientation.

Reminder:

In parenting, everything is connected! Our parenting decisions have ripple effects that connect beliefs and assumptions with our actions, and in turn our outcomes

Chapter 2

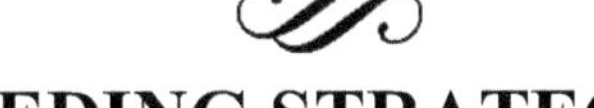

FEEDING STRATEGIES

Every decision made and every action taken as a result of our personal beliefs and assumptions sets in motion rippling effects of corresponding outcomes. Those outcomes are tied to the nature of our beliefs.

Feeding habits are essential to healthy sleep and infant care, and on the surface it sounds simple. Baby is hungry, so you feed. What else is there to know?

It's not that simple. How and when you feed have ripple effects across your baby's day, their sleep schedule, and in turn their development.

There are 3 major Feeding philosophies

1. Clock Feeding: Behaviorists in the 1900s emphasized environmental stimuli as the primary influence on human behavior, and downplayed the influence on internal factors like emotions and human will/nature. They believed if you could control the environmental influences, you could engineer the perfect child. They believed in a regimented feeding schedule every 4 hours - followed down to the minute. Baby's who were hungry outside these times were left to "cry it out". Because the clock determined when feedings occurred, it had little regard to the baby's immediate needs or the parent's natural intuition
2. Child-Led Feeding: Popularized in the 1940s through research done by Freud & Spock, suggested that labor and

delivery was so traumatizing to the unborn child that birth becomes a wellspring of mental imbalance and insecurity. To counteract this, mothers must "re-attach" to the baby emotionally. This theory holds two bizarre assumptions: one, that the womb is the perfect emotional relationship and attachment, an two, that the baby has a subconscious desire to return to the womb. Mothers were encouraged to endlessly cradle their babies, sleep with them, breast feed until the 3rd year, and that the child is to be the center of the family universe. What this actually produces is the opposite: emotionally-stressed, high-need, insecure babies and over-worked, endlessly tired mothers. While behaviorists emphasize outward structure and not inner person, the neo-primitivists emphasize the inner person at eh expense of any structure whatsoever. Bothare extreme and detrimental to healthy parenting. Parents should minister to the actual needs and vulnerabilities of their babies; however, they should be cautious of any parenting theory that creates extreme or false vulnerabilities. That is when healthy protection turns to unhealthy overprotection and long-term detriment.

3. **The Happy Baby Method - Parent Directed Feeding (PDF):** PDF is the center point between hyper-scheduling and re-attachment. It has enough structure to bring security and order, yet enough flexibility to give mom the freedom to respond to needs as they arise. it is proactive and helps foster healthy growth and optimal development. Embedded in the PDF strategy is a critical element for all aspects of infant care: Parental Assessment an acquired confidence to think, evaluate and intuitively learn what a baby needs & how to meet specific needs at specific times.

   A Baby cannot maximize learning without experiencing

optimal alertness. They can only experience optimal alertness with optimal sleep. Optimal sleep is created through good naps & established nighttime sleep. These sleeping patters are the end result of consistent feedings. Consistent feedings come from establishing a healthy routine.

Healthy routine = consistent feedings = optimal infant sleep = optimal alertness = optimal development

PDF eliminates the stress of relying exclusively on the variable of a hunger cue or the insufficient constant of the clock. In PDF, they are used together and backups to each other.

Hunger Cue + Clock + Parental Assessment = Feeding Time

you feed your baby when they are hungry, but the clock provides protective limits so you are not feeding too often or too little. PDF brings into play the critical tool of PA (Parental Assessment) to assess the baby's needs and respond accordingly. Here are some examples

PA provides tools to recognize and assess two potential problems with infant feeding:

1. The breast-fed child who feeds often - say every hour - may not be receiving adequate nutrition. Using PA, parents not only respond to the cue by feeding the baby, but are alerted to a potential problem with the feedings.
2. When the Hunger Cue is not present, the Clock serves as a guide to ensure that too much or too little time doesn't pass between feedings. It is also a protection for weak and sickly babies who may not be able to cry effectively.

3. When the hunger cue is present, the clock is secondary to the Cue because hunger, not the clock, determines feedings.

PDF & Comprehensive Attachment:

Comprehensive Attachment refers to the total spectrum of growth and development as measured by an infant's attainment of his or her developmental capacities. Infants who fail to attain these basic capacities within the first 6 months of life often become under-achievers in other developmental prerequisites leading to healthy relational attachment.

Babies are born with 7 capacities that when met, provide markers confirming Comprehensive Attachment is achieved. these markers are:

Synchronize their Feed-Wake-Sleep cycles into predictable patterns

1. Can fall asleep without rocking or nursing
2. Sleep through the night - 8-10hrs
3. Have a predictable nap routine
4. Content wake-times and are adapt to self-play
5. Able to self-soothe
6. Find comfort with other care-givers i.e. Fathers, siblings or grandparents

These markers are leading indicators the baby is not in a constant state of stress or anxiousness.

When these markers are not met - carrying on with 18 month or 2 year olds - it is a strong indicator of underdeveloped capacities and attachment deficits.

Chapter 3

BABIES & SLEEP

"You're so lucky"

"You've got an easy baby"

"Your baby is so happy! So content and alert."

These comments are not uncommon for PDF parents. But what does all this have to do with sleep? This is after all the #1 Baby SLEEP system right?

The answer is: Sleep has EVERYTHING to do with it.

Training your baby to sleep through the night is not the objective of parenting, but it provides a solid foundation for everything else that follows.

Sleep is one of the most significant influences on a healthy life. Sleep in the first year of life is not only critical to development, as growth hormones are released during sleep, but impacts the welfare of everyone else in the household. This separates happy, joyful parents from fatigued and often miserable ones.

FACT: Full- Term healthy babies are born with the capacity to sleep 7-8 hours at just 7-10 weeks old, and 10-12 hours of sleep by 12 weeks old.

Is this actually possible? Yes. Some babies are born sleepers (what we call low-need babies) and others are born waking easily & struggle (what we call high-need babies), but ALL babies can acquire the skill of sleeping through the night through parental training.

1. **RHYTHM:** Babies don't have the ability to organize their days & nights into predictable rhythms, but they have the biological need to do so. Parents must take the lead & create the valuable structure & routine for the baby and for themselves. The "feed-wake-sleep" routine is essential. The key to nighttime sleep lies in the order of those 3 daytime activities. They repeat themselves throughout the day, but the more consistent the routine, the faster the baby learns to adapt & adjust their rhythm to it. Established rhythms lead to continuous nighttime sleep
2. **FULL-FEEDING:** The quality of each step of the routine is just as important as the order. Make every feeding a FULL FEEDING. Babies (especially infants) are prone to dozing off while feeding, and only taking in a fraction of the nutrients they need. Particularly when breastfeeding, they are not ingesting enough nutrients to satisfy their needs. Keep them awake for a full feed before putting them to sleep. A full feed leads to a full nap which leads to full alertness & development during wake-times.
3. **HUNGER PATTERNS:** Baby hunger patterns tend to become erratic and unpredictable on their own, which is why infant hunger fed in the PDF system stabilizes.

    - Babies have an innate ability to organize their feeding times into a predictable rhythm, and will do so if encouraged by the mother.

- Digestion & Absorption respond to routine feedings with metabolic memory. Routine feedings incentives the hunger metabolism to organize into predictable cycles. Erratic or Cluster feedings discourage & confuse this process
- EX: Mom feeds her baby approximately every 3 hours: 7am, 10am, 1pm, 4pm, 7pm, 10pm. The baby's hunger cycle will synchronize with those established times. The principle to remember is consistency, not the times themselves. Start at 6, start at 10 it doesn't matter. Holding the consistency over time is what matters. Consistency = predictability.
- EX 2: Mom follows Cry-feeding method & suffers. 8am first feed, then 30min later then baby cries, then one hour later, then 4 hours later etc. No consistency leads to difficulty establishing Feed-Wake-Sleep rhythm & doesn't allow hunger metabolism to regulate. Her baby will most likely wake every 2 hours during the night and this pattern might last well into 24+ months of age.

4. **NOT WHAT, BUT WHEN:** There are debates about breastmilk vs. formula and when to use/stop using either. We did a study on 500 babies and found that when both raised in a PDF system, breastfed babies slept on average the same rates and sometimes sooner than formula-fed babies. This means the routine & rhythm are more

Deficits to unhealthy sleep include: diminished motor skills, decreased thinking capacity, irritability, loss of focusing ability, emotional instability, and cellular/tissue breakdown - and those are just the beginning!

As the higher brain develops during the first 2 years of life, the absence of continuous nights of sleep is detrimental to the learning process.

A 2 year old who cannot sleep through the night will be extremely prone to learning deficiencies & will potentially face life-long developmental issues.

Extended sleep is important, especially in the first year, as this is the time during which they experience rapid growth both physically & developmentally.

Healthy REM Cycle:

Babies alternate between quiet sleep and active sleep (RSP & ASP) around every 30 -45min. During quiet sleep the baby will be still and peaceful, during active sleep the arms & legs may stir, as well as the muscles in the face. It is important for babies to experience healthy cycles of each state for optimal development. This is achieved through extended nightly sleep.

A PDF STUDY:

Here are the statistical results of a study done observing the effects of the PDF system on 500 infants in 2016. 380 exclusively breastfed, 59 exclusively formula fed, 81 fed a combination of the two. 468 had no medical conditions & 32 with medical conditions detected at birth. 10 were premature infants. Routine feeding were established every 2.5-3hrs for the first 8 weeks. Nighttime sleep defined as 7+ continuous hours. Subjects were observed in the USA & Canada. The results were as follows:

1. **Exclusively Breastfed Infants:** 86.7% sleeping through the night between 7-8 weeks, 97% sleeping through the night by 12 weeks.
2. **Exclusively Formula-Fed Infants:** 82% sleeping through the night between 7-8 weeks, 96.4% sleeping through the night by 12 weeks
3. **Medical Condition Infants:** included reflux, colic, premature delivery, viral infections & unspecified hospitalizations. 100% slept 8+ hours between 13-16 weeks.

Got off to a bad start? No worries! On average across our studies, it only took 3-5 days for a 9 week old baby to break old patterns & acquire the skill of sleeping through the night!

Chronic fatigue in babies & young children is the primary cause of fussiness, irritability, crankiness, discontentment, colic symptoms, hypertension, bad focusing skills & bad eating habits.

Babies & young children with optimal rest are self-assured, happy, less demanding & more sociable. They have longer attention spans & as a result become fast-learners.

SLEEP PROPS

Our natural sleep cue is sleepiness, and sleep props interfere with the process by becoming a substitute cue for sleep instead of sleepiness. Some sleep props, like a special blanket or stuffed animal are harmless, while others can become addictive & harmful.

Here are those to avoid:

- **Intentionally nursing Baby to sleep** - obligating yourself to incessant nursing to put the baby down can be detrimental & disrupts the essential rhythm you are trying to establish. In the PDF system, babies are usually awake when they are placed in the crib. No tip-toeing or breath-holding needed. They may cry for a few minutes or talk to themselves, but they will fall asleep on their own without intervention from a parent
- **Motion & Vibration Props** - using a rocking chair or vibrating seat or something else is the fastest way to run out of patience as a parent. In the short & long run, putting the baby to bed while they are drowsy but awake facilitates longer & stronger sleep cycles than if placed in the crib when they are already asleep. They need to use sleepiness as their cue for sleep, not a ritual.
- **Sleeping With Your Baby** - while the co-sleeping trend is on the rise, not only is it extremely dangerous, since 2005 the AAP Task Force has determined that infant bed-sharing increases the risk of SIDS. Not only is the codependence counteractive to establishing a healthy PDF system, it is bad for their health.

Where should they sleep?

While the preference of a crib or bassinet can be debated, the more important thing to establish is where they sleep. Though having the baby share the room with the parents for the first 3 weeks may make nighttime feedings more convenient, but studies show room-sharing for 4 weeks can delay the baby's ability to sleep through the night for 4 months.

Put the baby in their own room & use a monitor to alert you to any immediate needs they have.

The best and safest way for your baby to fall asleep is the natural way. Confidently establish your basic PDF routine. Feed them, cradle & love them, put put them down in their crib before they fall asleep.

PUT THE TABLET DOWN!

It is a popular trend to distract & entertain babies & young children with games or videos on your tablet, phone, etc.

Devices emit Blue Light, which artificially stimulates the brain. Excessive exposure, especially at night, to blue light is directly linked to restless sleep, insomnia, anxiety, memory deficiencies, irritability, depression, stress, hypertension and unhealthy eating habits in ADULTS.

If the effects are that strong with adults, imagine what the effects are in Infants? Overloading your baby with artificial stimuli is detrimental to their development and will have irreversible life-long effects on their developmental abilities.

They may even become dependent on the stimuli and be unable to function without it i.e. unable to interact with other children/adults face to face, unable to interact in groups in a class room, & unable to learn & read.

A stimuli dependent baby/child is almost guaranteed to develop serious learning disabilities, unhealthy eating habits & emotional instability.

We have dealt with 8 year olds in our pediatric research who are unable to sleep through the night and still display underdeveloped Infantile behavior (crying when hungry, throwing tantrums when inconvenienced, etc.) and Autistic behavior (no eye contact, overly noise-sensitive, irritable, completely non-social, etc.) - despite not being on the Autism spectrum - due to their dependence on artificial blue light stimuli. Whatever initial potential they may have had, they are extremely cognitively under-developed to the point where they may never recover.

This is a serious issue facing parents nationwide.

It will be extremely difficult to establish a healthy sleep cycle when you are bombarding your infants developing brain with artificial stimuli.

Put the tablets down! We aren't saying don't use them at all or don't let your kids watch TV at all, but we are saying there need to be clear, monitored limits on how much blue light exposure they have, and there should be extremely little to none in the first 2 years of age.

Chapter 4

FEEDING FACTS

Breastmilk is the perfect food for babies. According to the AAP, breastmilk decreases incidence & severity of diarrhea, lower respiratory infections, bacterial meningitis, and UTIs. According to the AAP breastmilk also protects against SIDS, allergic diseases, Crohn's disease, ulcerative colitis, & other chronic digestive diseases. Breastmilk is easily digests and not only provides excellent nutrition, it also provides valuable antibodies for building the baby's immune system. Breastfeeding also benefits the mother by reducing risk of breast cancer, type 2 diabetes & osteoporosis later in life.

BREASTFEEDING TRENDS

According to the CDC, while 40% of new mothers begin exclusively breastfeeding, only 17% continue after 6 months.

Mothers following the PDF method have completely different statistics. A sample of 250 PDF mothers found that 88% of the mothers started breastfeeding, 80% exclusively (no formula/supplements), and while the national average dropped to 17% at 6 months, 70% of PDF mothers were exclusively breastfeeding.

The national average choses against the nourishment, convenience & closeness of breastfeeding primarily due to fatigue & endless demand created by a lack of routine & predictability in their home. Well-rested mothers with a predictable routine can focus on providing their babies with the best nutrients possible.

HUNGER CUES

Responding to hunger cue's are central to feeding, but where PDF feeding differs from cry-feeding is that PDF encourages full feedings about every 2.5-3hrs, rather than clusters of small feedings. Achieving full feedings is key to PDF success

Towards the end of a sleep cycle, the baby will often make little sucking sounds & may begin sucking on their hand. This might be followed with a soft whimper that can grow into a full cry. All those are cues its time to feed, but there is no need to wait until full-cry before feeding. Hunger cues always trump the time on the clock.

- unwelcome cues: EX: a baby nursing every hour may be a signal they are not receiving rich, high-calorie hindmilk, or not getting the quality of sleep needed. healthy sleep = healthy nursing = healthy growth. Fatigued babies do not nurse well & will want to nurse more often. The Mother's fatigue is another unwelcome cue. Continually waking exhausted means the mother's body is telling her what she is doing isn't working.

MILK PRODUCTION & FULL FEEDINGS

Breastfeeding is based on demand & supply. Supply of milk is proportional to demand placed on the body. Adequate demand produces adequate supply - but how do we define these?

A mother who breastfeeds 12-20 times/day will not

necessarily produce more milk than a mother who breastfeeds 8-10 times/day. The difference is in the quality of the feedings. PDF babies take fewer feedings, but they are full feedings. Routine-less mothers may feed constantly but they are partial & incomplete feedings.

Whether breast or bottle feeding, a full-feed is what to aim for.

What characteristics are common with a full feed?

obvious ones are:

1. minimum 10-15min per breast, or 20-30min for formula-fed babies
2. Hearing the baby swallow the milk
3. The baby pulling away from the breast or bottle when full
4. Burping well after feeding
5. Napping well after feeding

Infants fed on a 2.5-3hr routine have a stable digestive metabolism & demand more milk during a feeding than babies who periodically feed throughout the day.

MOM CARE

While it is important to maintain a balanced, healthy diet; don't forget to hydrate! Mothers should drink 6- 8 ounces of water at or around each feeding (this can also include juice, broth & tea). This does not include coffee & black tea (diuretics that will dehydrate you), and Sodas (high in chemicals, sugar & sodium).

LET-DOWN REFLUX

When a baby begins to suckle, 2 hormones are released in the mother's body: Prolactin & Oxytocin. Prolactin is necessary for milk production & oxytocin for release. At the beginning of the feed, the baby receives foremilk, milk stored in ducts directly behind the nipple, which has little nutritional value. As the suckling continues, the oxytocin contracts the glands forcing milk into the ducts. This sensation is known as "let-down reflux". This milk is called hind milk, which is the high calorie, high protein, high fat milk that is necessary for baby growth & development.

BREASTMILK & DIGESTION

Though breastmilk digests faster than formula, this doesn't mean breastfed babies need to feed more often. An empty stomach is not what triggers hunger, it is completed absorption in the body that signals for hunger. A drop in blood sugar is what triggers hunger, not an empty stomach.

Therefore, efficient feedings will provide maximum nutrition absorption and therefore less frequent feedings.

FEEDING HYGIENE

Wash hands with soap & water before feeding. Hand sanitizers kill all non-porous bacteria including many healthy bacteria that live on your skin.

PROPER NURSING POSITIONS

Uncomfortable neck position leads to difficult feedings. Align your baby's body for maximum feeding efficiency.

There are 3 interchangeable nursing positions:

1. **Cradle:** While sitting, place your baby's head in the curve of your arm. A pillow under your arm will lessen the stress on your neck & upper back. Remember to keep the Baby's body properly aligned & facing your breasts.
2. **Side-Lying:** Often used by mothers recovering from Cesarean births. Both Mother and baby lie facing each other, with the baby supported by a pillow. The baby's head should be centered on the breast.
3. **Football Hold:** One hand under the baby's head while lifting & supporting the breast with the other. Center the nipple on the baby's mouth & stroke lightly downward toward the lower lip.

HOW OFTEN TO FEED?

In the beginning, every 2.5-3hrs (may be slightly less or more depending on your hunger cues). Time between feedings is measured as the time from the beginning of a feed to the beginning of the next. The time it takes for a full feed (approx. 20-30min), total wake and sleep time averages 2hrs, so you have your 2.5-3hr Feed-Wake-Sleep cycle.

NAP TIMES

It is easy to assume the longer the better, but in a healthy PDF system, you should feed every 2.5-3hrs with 1.5-2hr nap times. Just like you don't want to go too long or too short between feeds, it is important for naps to not go too long or too short. If they sleep too long, wake them up! Establishing your routine is what will produce longer nighttime sleeps. You want to stay as close to the 2.5-3hr cycle range as possible in the first few weeks.

3 MILK PHASES

1. Colostrum: 5x higher in protein. Has rich antibodies that protect the baby from a variety of bacterial & viral illnesses. It also facilitates the meconium stool - the first stool a baby passes.
2. Transition Milk: begins within 2-4 days and lasts 7-14 days. Less protein than Colostrum & increase in fat, calories & vitamins.
3. Mature milk: comprised of foremilk & followed several minutes into a feed by hindmilk. Thinner consistency, higher calorie content.

Feed Rhythm

With Colostrum, much thicker than Mature Milk, the pattern is usually suck, suck, suck, swallow. When Mature Milk begins to flow, your baby responds with a healthy suck, swallow, suck, swallow, etc. At this point hard sucking is reduced as should tenderness in the breast.

NURSING CHALLENGES IN THE FIRST 10 DAYS

1. The first Nursing: Most babies are alert for the first 90min after birth, making it the ideal time to begin nursing. Initially begin 10-15min each side for sufficient breast stimulation.
2. Sleepy Newborns: After Postpartum alertness, babies love sleep. Newborns need to feed every 2-3hrs, so asleep or not they need to eat. Also to achieve a full feed, you need to keep the baby awake until a full feed is done.
3. Birth Weight: Babies are born with additional fluids &

the meconium stool, so after these pass the baby will appear to lose weight (most babies 5-7% of their birth weight). Don't be alarmed, know & compare their birth weight with their weight at the time of hospital discharge. After this initial drop in weight, you will see them put weight back on relatively quickly.

4. Measuring Food Intake: What should you look for? 5-7 wet diapers/day the first week, 3-5 more yellow stools daily for the first month, & consistent weight gain are good signs the baby is receiving enough milk for optimal growth & development
5. First 7-10 Days: You will ease into the PDF 2.5-3hr cycle soon enough, in the first 7-10 days, focus primarily on achieving a full feed every time you nurse. Nursings for the first 14 days may average 30-40min per feed (These figures are statistical averages, not guarantees). If you can achieve full feedings during your first 14 days, the transition into the PDF system is quite natural within 2 weeks
6. How Long to Nurse? Some nurse 15-20min on one side, burp, then offer the other side for another 15-20min. Some Mothers offer each breast for 10min, burping in-between sides, and then offering each breast for an additional 5min. Either is fine, the second method is helpful with sleepy baby as the disruptions will help them stay awake.

GROWTH SPURTS

What if your baby is hungrier sooner than 2.5hrs? Even with full feedings, when a baby hits a growth spurt, they might need additional feedings. They can last 1-4 days, and after everything returns to normal.

Are Growth Spurts predictable? Not exactly. Generally they are believed to happen 10 days after birth followed by 3 weeks, 6 weeks, 3 months & 6 months. Timing varies from baby to baby but if you notice sudden hunger increase around these times, it is most likely a growth spurt. Typical other signs are waking 40-50min early from a nap extremely hungry & this cycle repeats every 2hrs.

How do you know when it is over? Growth Spurts are just as tiring for the baby as they are for the mother, when the normal cycle resumes, the baby will nap longer than normal.

BREASTMILK VS. FORMULA

When it comes to nutritional value, babies thrive on both. In the broader benefits, breastmilk is superior - especially in the first 12 weeks. Between 6-12 months the gap between the two decreases considerably.

Breastfeeding past a year is unnecessary, and other foods will have been introduced into the baby's diet by then as well.

While we encourage breastfeeding, we realize not all moms can or will. Your decision to breast or bottle feed is not a negative or positive judgement on your motherhood, nor will it emotionally impact the baby.

BOTTLE FEEDING

Most important is to those the right-sized hole. Too large forces the baby to drink too fast & can lead to spitting up & vomiting. Too small the baby can't get enough & will stay hungry. the test: hold the bottle upside down. There should be a slow drip of formula.

FORMULA

Cow's milk is not suitable for children under 1 year old.

How much formula? 2.5 ounces for each pound of body weight i.e. 16lb baby should get 36oz of formula in a 24hr period. Once the baby is sleeping through the night, this means 6-8oz every 3-4hrs. Do not exceed the 2.5oz/1lb weight portion unless directed so by your pediatrician.

Do not bottle feed while baby is lying flat, this may lead to ear infection & tooth decay.

BURPING THE BABY

Gently pat your way up the baby's back.

Burping Positions:

Sitting Lap: Place hand over Baby's stomach. Hook thumb around side of baby while wrapping the rest of your fingers around the chest. Lean the baby slightly forward & begin.

Tummy-Over-Lap: While sitting, place baby's legs between your legs & drape the baby over your thigh. While supporting the head with your hand, bring your knees together & begin.

1. Shoulder Position: With baby's chest resting on a cloth high on your shoulder, begin.
2. Cradle Position: Cradle baby with bottom in hand & head resting at your elbow. One arm & one leg are to be wrapped around her arm, making sure the baby is facing away from her. Begin

SPITTING UP & PROJECTILE VOMITING

When air bubbles are trapped during feeding, they release some of the ingested milk when they are released by the burp. Spitting up is fairly common, and usually signals the stomach has taken slightly more than it can handle. No need to be worried, but monitor how often it happens. If consistent, reduce the oz the baby is receiving. Projectile vomiting is rare and not an issue, however if you experience routine episodes, it may indicate a more serious problem: Gastroesophageal Reflux and/or also intestinal infection. Establishing correct diagnosis & treatment is very important.

BURPING CHALLENGES

With newborns, if after trying for 5min, place them in an infant seat rather than the crib. Gravity will help keep the milk down & the air bubbles up. placing the infant in a seat for 10-15min is helpful preventing milk from refluxing into the esophagus.

HICCUPS

Even if you are doing everything perfect, there will be times when air bubbles are trapped in the stomach or intestine, resulting in hiccups. To alleviate baby's discomfort, place them in a knee-chest position with their back next to your chest & pull their knees up to their chest. They usually last 5-30min.

BOTH ENDS

Healthy stools indicate healthy feeding & growth. Early on baby will have bowel movements after each feeding, or at least several times/day. Frequent stools are a sign everything is working efficiently.

5-7 wet diapers daily are signs that your baby is receiving adequate milk for growth. After 4 weeks, stool pattern decreases from several/day to one or two/day. It is also not uncommon for exclusively breastfed babies to go several days without a bowel movement around 8 weeks.

Chapter 5

YOUR BABY'S DAY

How do you establish a baby's routine that is predictable, but flexible enough to meet the growing & changing Feed-Wake-Sleep needs?

Something that is flexible is something that can be bent or pulled but return to its original shape. You must first establish a routine on which your flexibility will be based. This way after a growth spurt or a sickness etc. your baby will snap back into their routine.

Sample Infant Routine Schedule Weeks 1-2:

7am	1. Feed, Diaper Change, Hygiene Care 2. Waketime: Minimal 3. Down for nap
9:30am	1. Feed, Diaper Change, Hygiene Care 2. Waketime: Minimal 3. Down for nap
12pm	1. Feed, Diaper Change, Hygiene Care 2. Waketime: Minimal 3. Down for nap
2:30pm	1. Feed, Diaper Change, Hygiene Care 2. Waketime: Minimal 3. Down for nap
5pm	1. Feed, Diaper Change, Hygiene Care 2. Waketime: Minimal 3. Down for nap
8pm	1. Feed, Diaper Change, Hygiene Care 2. Waketime: Minimal 3. Down for nap
11pm	Feed, diaper change, down for sleep. Allow Baby to wake naturally but don't let them sleep longer than 4 hours continuously for the first 4 weeks
1:30am	Feed, Diaper Change & right back to bed
4am	Feed, Diaper Change & right back to bed

Sample Routine Schedule Weeks 48-52:

7:30am	1. Feed 2. Waketime activities 3. Down for nap
11:30am	1. Feed 2. Watetime activities 3. Down for nap
3:30-4pm	1. Snack after nap 2. Waketime activity 3. Dinner time with family 4. Early evening wake time
8pm	Down for the night

The 3 activities in the baby's routine are Feeding Time, Wake Time and Naptime. The challenge for parents is knowing when the changes are coming & how they should respond.

1. Walk a year's worth of changes in the routine & talk about when they come & how you adjust the cycle.
2. Review the guidelines associated with the Routine activities for the first 12 weeks
3. Introduce principles that will govern the Routines.

Merging - Parental Management is all about merging the changing needs of one growth stage to the next.

Compare the routine schedule differences between 1-2 week old vs. a 10-12month old:

Sample Infant Routine Schedule Weeks 1-2:

One by one, the cycles merged as the baby develops. 9 cycles to 8, 8 to 7, etc. until just 3.

At this point there are 3 pressing questions:

1. What changes can parents expect?
2. When can parents expect them (average)?
3. What adjustments will parents have to make?

Every baby is different when it comes to timing, but we know the average times when cycles begin to merge.

Typically Babies begin with 9-10 cycles, and should be at 3 by week 52, so just as important as when the merges happen is how many merges there are. Here are some guidelines that can help to navigate the various cycle merges (average PDF babies have 7 merges).

1. Capacity & Ability: A mother can't arbitrarily decide to skip a feeding or change nap time
2. unless the baby has the physical capacity and ability to make the adjustment. EX: 2 week old cannot go 8 hours with food or sleep through the night, so the mother shouldn't be thinking about dropping a night feed.
3. Time Variation: While the length of each cycle remains consistent early on, eventually each
4. cycle will take on its own features. EX: for a 4mo baby, 1 cycle might be as short as 2.5hrs, while another might be 3.5hrs (remember, no cycle should be longer than 4hrs & no shorter than 2. Ideally 2.5-3hrs max). At 6mo, everything changes again. The range variation depends on the baby's age, unique needs & time of day.
5. First-Last Feeding: No matter which Merge is taking

place, the first feed of the day is ALWAYS the most strategic and important when adjusting the routine. While there can be some flexibility to the first feed time, try to keep it within a 20min time frame. Flexibility comes after routine is established. The consistency will also help Mom plan her day around feeding & napping times. After your baby is sleeping through the night 8+ hrs, the first & last feeds become the most strategic as the whole cycle of the day will be set with these parameters.

6. Individuality: All experience the same merges, but perhaps not at the same time. EX cousins John & Emily. John started sleeping through the night at 6 weeks, Emily began sleeping through the night at 10 weeks (4 week difference). At 12 Weeks, Emily is sleeping 12hrs, and John never sleeps longer than 10hrs his whole first year. They both experienced the same 2 merges - dropping middle-of-the-night & late-evening feeds - but at different, though still relative, times and according to their individual needs.
7. **Two steps forward, one step back:** It can only take a day to adopt a new pattern, but most merges take 4-6 days to establish. EX: week 6 your baby sleeps 6hrs, week 7 up to 7hrs, then for 4 days, they only sleep 5hrs. Eventually they get over 8+ hours. This is common during various merges. Allow 4-6 days for your baby to adjust.

All of these guidelines work for both bottle & breast fed babies.

Principle to Practice

What are the developmental "triggers" signaling its time to

merge cycles? For PDF babies, most triggers are predictable & fall into a chronological range of time.

7 major triggers for the 7 major merges over the course of the first year.

MERGE 1: 3-6 weeks

Most babies start out with 2 middle of the night feeds EX 2 & 5am. Sometime between 3-6 weeks, PDF babies begin to stretch their middle of the night sleep from 3-3.5-4hrs. They naturally begin to merge the 2am & 5am Feeds into a single 3am feed.

2am feed

week 3-4 merge to 3am feed

5am feed

This is the first merge, from 9 cycles to 8. Sleeping 4-hour stretches become the new normal.

MERGE 2: 7-10 weeks

Turing this time most Happy Baby Method babies drop the middle of the night feeding & begin sleeping 8hrs. 8 cycles now become 7. Your baby won't be eating less, they will just be taking in more calories during each feed.

*At 5 weeks, most babies can extend nighttime sleep by 1 hour each week. A healthy 5 week old can handle a 5hr stretch at night, a 7 week old can handle a 7hr stretch at night.

Adjustment to Baby's Routine after Merge 2: Once the baby merges the 'middle of the night' feeds, make some adjustments to the daytime routine. Before the baby made it through the night, Mom was feeding every 3hrs, which fit into a 24hr routine.

Now that the baby is sleeping through the night, the original math doesn't work anymore (24hrs - 8hrs sleep = 16hrs & we need to fit in 7 feedings, which works out to every 2.5hrs not 3+)

1. Decide the time for the morning feed. It doesn't matter whether you keep the original time or not, but a defined time needs to be established. Remember, the later you have the first morning feed, the later it pushes the last feed.
2. Based on this time, schedule 7 Feeds for the day
3. Remember the first-last principle. When reworking a Baby's routine, you must fit the other five Feed-Wake-Sleep cycles between the first morning feed & the last evening feed. Though they keep an even structure, they don't have to be equal in length. Every parent must decide for themselves what works best for their baby.

Challenges:

- **Busy Schedules:** Busy Moms often experience lower milk supply (quantity & quality) during the late afternoon. Because of this, she will have to offer the early-evening feed within 2hrs of the previous feed
- **Growth Spurts:** Will also require temporary, sooner-

than-normal feeds

- When late evening feed is between 8:30pm-midnight, some Moms prefer to feed at 8:30pm & again at 10:30pm, so that Mom can go to bed earlier while not disturbing the Baby's nighttime sleep.

Sample Schedule after Merge 2 (Weeks 7-10)

Early Morning 6:30-7am

1. Feed, Diaper Change, Hygiene Care
2. Waketime
3. Nap

Mid-Morning 9:30am

1. Feed, Diaper Change, Hygiene Care
2. Waketime
3. Nap

Midday 12:30pm

1. Feed, Diaper Change, Hygiene Care
2. Waketime
3. Nap

Mid-Afternoon 3:30pm

1. Feed, Diaper Change, Hygiene Care
2. Waketime
3. Nap

Late Afternoon 5:30-6pm

1. Feed, Diaper Change, Hygiene Care
2. Waketime
3. Nap

Early Evening 8-8:30pm	1.	Feed, Diaper Change, Hygiene Care
	2.	Nap
Late Evening 10:30-11pm	1.	Feed, Diaper Change, Hygiene Care
	2.	Sleep for the Night

MERGE 3: BETWEEN WEEKS 10-15

This is when most Happy Baby Method/PDF babies drop their Late Evening feed & begin sleeping 10-12hrs through the night.

When this happens, 7 Cycles becomes 6 Cycles.

The morning feed remains the same, the baby will simply drop the last feed cycle of the day & go down for the night at 8-8:30pm.

This new phase continues until the Baby starts to eat solid foods, between 4.5-6 months old

Sample Schedule After Merge 3: Weeks 10-15

Early Morning 6:30-7am	1. Feed 2. Wake 3. Nap
Mid-morning 9:30am	1. Feed 2. Wake 3. Nap
Mid Day 12:30pm	1. Feed 2. Wake 3. Nap
Mid-Afternoon 3:30pm	1. Feed 2. Wake 3. Nap
Late Afternoon 5:30-6pm	1. Feed 2. Wake 3. Nap

Evening 8:30-9pm

1. Feed
2. Sleep For the Night

Challenge for breastfeeding: When still breastfeeding, remember milk production. Allowing the baby to sleep 10+hrs may not provide enough stimulation in a 24hr period to maintain adequate supply. While not the case for all breastfeeding moms, this particularly impacts breastfeeding Moms in their mid- 30s or older. In this case, we recommend keeping the Late Evening feed, between 10:30-11pm until Week 16

MERGE 4: BETWEEN WEEKS 16-24

During this time, most PDF babies begin to extend the morning wake time by merging the early morning & mid-morning feeds. This brings our Cycles from 6 to 5. Lunchtime is usually moved up at least 30min so there is only 1 Feed-Wake-Sleep cycle between Morning & Lunch.

This is also close to the time when solid foods start becoming necessary. This can impact the timing of activities. During this phase, there is no more full-nap between the Late Afternoon & Evening Feeds, just perhaps a 30-40min "catnap"

Sample Schedule after Merge 4 (Weeks 16-24)

Morning 7am	1. Feeding 2. Waketime 3. Nap
Late Morning	1. Feeding 2. Waketime 3. Nap
Early Afternoon	1. Feeding 2. Waketime 3. Nap

Late Afternoon

- Feeding
- Waketime
- *possible Catnap

Evening 8-8:30pm	1. Early Evening Waketime 2. Liquid Feed, Sleep for the Night

The Times of the 3 during-the-day Cycles after this Merge are somewhat flex. It is important to have established Morning & Evening Feed times, but the other times are flexible with the baby's development & digestion. Example: 7am, 11am, 2pm, 5pm, 8pm. Baby's with longer Early Afternoon Naps may have times like 7am, 10am, 1pm, 5:30pm, 8pm.

MERGE 5: BETWEEN WEEKS 24-39

Between 5-7 months

Introduction of solid foods & the emergence of the "catnap"

Catnaps range between 30 minutes - 1 hr and happen usually around dinnertime in the late afternoon.

Going from full-nap to catnap doesn't eliminate a Feed-Wake-Sleep cycle, but it moves in that direction.

PDF babies typically drop their 3rd naps & move to catnaps between 24-39 weeks. This large time frame represents huge variation among babies, yet is a normal range of predictable behavior.

Once your baby drops their 3rd full-nap, the Feed-Wake-Sleep cycles range between 3.5 - 4.5hrs (this depends on unique needs & time of day).

Sample Schedule After Merge Five (Weeks 24-39)

Morning 7am	1. Feeding 2. Waketime 3. Nap
Late Morning 11am	1. Feeding 2. Waketime 3. Nap

Mid-Afternoon 3pm

1. Feeding
2. Waketime
3. Cat-Nap

Late Afternoon/Dinnertime 7pm	1.Feeding 2.Waketime
Early Evening 8-8:30pm	1.Waketime 2.Liquid Feed, Sleep for night

*Remember, first & last times matter most. The 3 in the middle are subjected/based on your individual & unique baby needs & timeframe you choose

MERGE 6: BETWEEN WEEKS 28-40

Sometime in this phase, PDF babies drop their catnap, reducing the Five cycles to Four, requiring more daytime adjustments. The 4 Cycles include: Breakfast, Lunch, Dinner &

a liquid feed at bedtime.

Some babies might drop the catnap at 31 weeks while others until 39 weeks, but both are within the normal range. It should happen between weeks 28-40, but when is up to your baby's individual, unique needs.

During this phase babies begin to receive cereal, vegetables, or fruits in the late afternoon meal can begin joining the rest of the family in eating with light finger foods (More of a snack than a full meal).

Sample Schedule After Merge Six: Weeks 28-40

Breakfast 7-8am	1. Feeding 2. Waketime 3. Nap
Mid-Day	1. Feeding 2. Waketime 3. Nap

Late Afternoon

- Feeding
- Waketime
- Dinner with Family (Snack)
- Early evening waketime

Bedtime 8pm

1. Liquid feeding, sleep for night

MERGE 7: BETWEEN WEEKS 46-52

Congratulations! You've made if from 9 Cycles to 4

During this phase, your baby no longer receives a liquid feeding before bed. They might receive a cup of formula, breastmilk, or juice, but a bottle of milk is not necessary.

Sample Schedule After Merge Seven: Weeks 46-52

Breakfast 7am	1. Feeding 2. Waketime 3. Nap
Mid-Day	1. Feeding 2. Waketime 3. Nap

Late Afternoon 4-5pm

- After Nap Snack
- Waketime
- Dinner Time with Family
- Early evening Waketime

Bedtime 8pm

1. Sleep for Night

SPECIFIC FEEDING AND WAKE-TIME GUIDELINES

Specific & Helpful Reminders Feeding and the First Twelve Weeks

1. During the first week, stay mindful that newborns are

prone to snacking. A series of snack feedings do not add up to full feedings! Your Baby needs to eat and the breastfeeding mom needs the stimulation that comes with full-feeds.

2. For Newborns, all of the waketime activities: feeding, burping, diaper change, etc. will be approx. 30min. The following Nap should be 1.5-2hrs maximum. The entire initial Feed-Wake-Sleep Cycle should average 2.5hrs.
3. Around 3 weeks, baby will begin to extend their waketime after each feed. This will extend to 30min beyond feeding. On average, waketime is followed by a 1.5-2hr nap
4. At 6 weeks, feed times are still approx. 30min & wake times begin to increase 30-50min, followed by a 1.5-2hr nap. By 12 weeks, wake times could be a full 60min or more.

How to Merge/Drop Feeds

Babies drop feeds because they are sleeping longer or staying awake longer. Dropping a feed requires adjustments to the daily routine that babies often need help with. this is where the collective wisdom of experienced mothers comes in handy.

Here are a few time-tested suggestions to consider:

1. **Dropping the middle of the night feed** - between 7-10 weeks, most PDF babies drop this feed on their own. One night they simply sleep til morning. Though PDF babies have the capacity and ability to make this adjustment, sometimes they may need a little nudge because their

internal sleep clock is “stuck”. You will know this is occurring if they wake within 5min of the same time each night for 3 nights in a row. How to handle this:

- Allow Baby to Resettle on their Own - Aside from the usual monitoring & periodically checking on the baby, simply patting them on the back & letting them know you are there will be enough to allow the baby to learn to resettle themselves. Normally after 3-4 nights with some crying, the internal sleep clock adjusts & the baby begins sleeping through until morning.
- Push late-evening feed closer to 11pm or midnight - Once the baby is sleeping through the night, you can gradually back up the late-evening feeds by 15-30min increments until the last feed of the day is where you want it to be.
- The Backward Slide (Last Resort) - EX: if your baby wakes up at 3am, preempt this ritual by waking them up and feeding them 15-30min earlier, in this example, 2:30-45am. If they then sleep till normal morning wake time, in a couple of days begin trying to move the time back 30-60min each night (2:30am, 2:00am, 1:30am, 1:00am, etc.) until the late-night feed time becomes a time you are comfortable with & establishing as your last feed time of the day.

2. **Dropping the Late-Evening Feed** - Occurs at around 3months of age & is usually the trickiest feed to eliminate. Once you get used to sleeping all night, some parents are hesitant to drop the late-evening feed out of

the fear that this will cause the baby to begin waking up in the middle of the night. If your baby is showing a lack of interest or is difficult to wake up for this feed, those are good signs they are ready to drop the feed. The way to drop this feed is by gradually adjusting the other feed times.

- EX: If the late-afternoon feed is around 6pm, try feeding the baby again at 9:30pm for a few days, then move the feed to 9:15 or 9pm for the next two days. Continue gradually adjusting the time backward until you reach your desired bedtime for the baby to sleep through the night. Dropping this feed will often make the last two feeds less than 3hrs apart. This should not be a problem, as the last feed of the day is the priority in this case.

SLEEP GUIDELINES & THE 1ST MONTH

Waking up a sleeping baby for feeds: When should you wake a sleeping baby & when should you let them sleep?

If you need to wake them up during the day to prevent them sleeping longer than the 3hr cycle, do it. Such intervention is necessary to stabilize the baby's digestive metabolism & help organize their sleep patterns into a predictable routine.

The one exception comes with late-evening & middle of the night feeds. During the 1st month a baby may give parents a 4hr stretch of sleep at night - but don't let them sleep longer than 4hrs. Wake them up, feed them & put them right back to bed - an infant under 4wks is too young to go longer without food.

WAKETIME & THE 1ST 3 MONTHS

In the first 2wks, your baby will not have a distinct wake time apart from feeding. This is all a newborn can handle before they need to sleep again. Usually by weeks 2-3, babies fall into a predictable feed-wake-sleep cycle.

Once you make it through the first few weeks, life begins to settle as your routine takes shape.

What might a FWS routine look like in the first 2 weeks?

BIRTH-2 WEEKS

Feed Time/Waketime	Sleep
30-50min	1.5-2hrs

———————2-3hrs———————

Remember, during this phase, wake time is almost indistinguishable from Feed time, this slightly changes in weeks 3-5

3-5 WEEKS

Feed Time Waketime	Sleep
30-60min	1.5-2hrs

———————2.5-3hrs———————

At this stage, wake time begins to separate from Feed time, lasting up to 30min. (not that it should be 30min, but up to 30min in addition to feed time).

You will see a new level of alertness begin to emerge at this stage & beginning around week 6, wake time becomes more distinct & feed time more precise:

6-12 WEEKS

Feed Time	Waketime	Sleep
30min	30-50min	1.5-2hrs

————————————————2.5-3.5hrs————————————————-

By week 12, wake times could be 60min or longer. By then your baby should be slccping through the night.

As wake time begins to lengthen there is potential for a subtle and not ideal shift in the cycle routine that must be avoided at all cost. Do not allow a wake-feed-sleep order to overtake the established feed-wake-sleep routine order!

It can happen easily: Mom is feeding 7wk old, but today the baby falls asleep without an adequate waketime. After a shorter than normal nap, Baby wakes & isn't interested in feeding because they aren't hungry yet. Trying to stay on schedule, Mom then waits to feed 20-30min. Instead of feeding after the nap when they are well rested, baby is now feeding after a wake time when they have less energy to feed efficiently.

This isn't an issue if it happens once or twice, but it is critical that you do not allow this to become routine.

Inadequate waketimes = insufficient sleep = shorter naps = inefficient feeds = cycle chaos

Feeds should follow directly after naps in the early months.

GENERAL GUIDELINES: CONTEXT!

Examples of PDF flexibility and how context of situation is

important

1. 2wk old is unceremoniously woken up by older sibling. Sibling tells Mom baby is crying. It is another 30min before the next scheduled feed - what does she do? She can:
    1. Try resettling the baby by patting them on the back or holding them
    2. Placing them in a bouncy seat
    3. Feed them now & rework the next Feed-Wake-Sleep cycle to space the rest of the day out correctly.
2. You are in an airplane & infant begins to fuss loudly. She just ate an hour ago, what do you do?
    1. Don't allow your routine to override being thoughtful to others. If attempts to play with & entertain the baby fail, go ahead & feed them, for the context of the situation dictates the temporary hold of your normal routine. Once you arrive, make the appropriate adjustments to the rest of the day schedule.
3. You just fed baby before dropping them off at the nursery & are planning to return in 90min. Should you leave a bottle of breastmilk or formula just in case?
    1. Yes! Nursery Workers (& babysitters) provide a valuable service, but since their care covers other children as well, they should not be obligated to follow your routine to the minute. If your baby makes a fuss, they should have the option of offering a bottle. Receiving early feedings a few times/week will not ruin a well-established routine

4. You have been in the car for 4hrs & it is your normal feed time, but baby is asleep & you only have another 30min to drive. You can:

   a) Choose to pull over & feed baby
   b) Just wait until you arrive & adjust the rest of the day's cycles accordingly.

Most days will be routine & predictable, but life happens, and there will be times when flexibility is needed. Life will be less tense if you understand the context of your situations & respond appropriately.

SLEEP & NAP SUMMARY YEAR 1

WEEKS	TIME SPENT SLEEPING	NUMBER OF NAPS/DAY
1-2	17-19hrs	5-6
3-5	16-18hrs	5-6
6-7	15-18hrs	4-6
8-12	14-17hrs	4-5
13-15	13-17hrs	3-4
16-24	13-16hrs	3-4
25-38	13-15hrs	2-3
39-52	12-15hrs	2

Chapter 6

When Baby Cries

All Babies cry, often without any apparent cause. Newborns routinely cry a total of 1-4 hours a day. No mother can console her child every time they cry, so do not expect to be a miracle worker with your baby. Pay close attention to your baby's different cries & you'll soon be able to tell when he needs to be picked up, consoled, or tended to, and when they are better off left alone.

Think of crying as a signal, not a statement against your parenting or a reaction to pain, fear, or discomfort.

Here are some cries & possible solutions:

Crying immediately after a feed:

If baby cries routinely within 30min after a feed, and it sounds like a pain cry more than a sleepy cry, it may be because of these three factors:

1. **Trapped Gas** - Young babies & Infants often swallow air during feeds. This is what makes post-feed burping so important. Trapped Gas is the first cause to blame when a baby wakes up 30min into a nap. This cry is often a high-pitched scream. If you find yourself in this situation, simply burp the baby and cuddle them for a moment before putting them back down to continue sleeping.
2. **Your Diet (Mom)** - If breastfeeding, consider what you

are eating. Avoid large quantities of dairy products & spicy foods.

3. **Milk-Quality Issues -** It is possible to have sufficient quantity of breastmilk but not enough quality. If this is the issue, your baby will respond with a hunger cry within an hour. Although rare, this affects 5% of nursing mothers. What can you do? Check your diet & consult your pediatrician. They may recommend a nutritionist.

Crying in the middle of a nap: If your baby abruptly wakes up with a strong cry, it may be a cause of the 3 previously listed factors or their sleep schedule was disrupted the previous evening or a hectic morning. It may also be the cause of **Nap Challenges:**

Nap Challenges:

1. Baby is hungry because:
    1. Did not have a full-feed in last feed
    2. Baby needs more milk calories in 24-hr period
    3. Baby is starting a growth spurt
    4. Baby is ready to start solid foods

2. Baby is uncomfortable because:
    1. Baby is getting sick, has slight fever, is teething, is starting an ear infection
    2. Baby has an insect bit or hair twisted around a toe (tourniquet syndrome)
    3. Baby is too hot or too cold
    4. Baby has diaper rash

3. Baby's stomach is upset because:
    3. Baby has mild or delayed case of reflux

4. Baby is having an allergic reaction to a new baby food
5. Baby is struggling with a bowel movement
6. Baby needs to burp

4. Baby woke up because:
   1. Baby startled themselves
   2. Baby rolled over & does not know how to roll back (very common)
   3. Baby lost pacifier & cannot resettle without it

5. Baby is starting a sleep/nap transition because:
   1. Baby is extending nighttime sleep, affecting daytime naps
   2. Baby's body does not require as much sleep in a 24hr period, impacting naps

Sleep Challenges related to Mom

1. Baby is hungry because
2. 1. The previous feed proved to be inadequate
3. 2. Mom's milk supply has decreased
4. Mom's diet is affecting the nursing baby
5. Baby has a reaction to medication Mom is taking
6. Nursing baby is getting too much lactose from Mom
7. Mom's schedule was rushed, so she did not allow enough time for baby to get a full feed

Sleep challenges related to activities

1. Previous waketime was too short
2. Previous waketime was over-stimulating because
   1. Waketime was too long, promoting fatigue rather than sleepiness

2. Waketime activity was too over-stimulating (ex: exposure to Blue Light from devices)
3. Baby's routine has too much flexibility (Ex: Mom running too many errands & Baby catnapping in car in-between stops)
4. First Feed of the day has too much flexibility in scheduling
5. Cycle out of order. Baby on Wake-Feed-Sleep schedule instead of Feed-Wake-Sleep

Sleep Challenges related to the Environment

1. Baby not being exposed to enough daylight. Natural light helps babies regulate their circadian clock
2. Baby's room not dark enough for nap/sleep time
3. Baby is over-stimulated in the crib with loud or electronic toys
4. When baby is 4-6mo, they could be waking up in response to familiar sounds in the home (dishwasher, laundry machine, parents voices, etc.)
5. Unknown Reasons: What does this mean? Simply that no clear reason exists, but it is unique to your baby's situation & that is not seen in many other babies

Normal Crying

Crying just before feeding - in normal circumstances, this crying is very short as the next event in the baby's cycle is feeding. If baby is hungry, feed them. If they routinely show signs of hunger before the next feed, find out why instead of letting them cry it out. Your baby's routine is to serve you and your baby, not vise versa.

Crying during the Late-Afternoon/Early-Evening period - Most babies have a “fussy time”, especially in the Late-Afternoon. Literally millions of parents are going through the same thing every day. If your baby is not comforted by a baby swing, an infant seat, siblings, or grandparent, consider the crib. At least there they have the chance of falling asleep. If your baby is exceptionally & continuously fussy, consider the possibility that they are hungry. How is milk supply? How is your diet?

*Challenges with crying related to colic, reflux & other issues are covered in the next Module

Crying when going down for a Nap - Duration of crying is set by the baby but monitored by the parent. According to the AAP, this is not a sign their basic needs are not being met but that babies have a natural disposition to cry before sleeping. According to AAP research, many babies cannot fall asleep without crying & will go to sleep more quickly if left to cry for a while. Crying should not last long if the child is truly tired (15 minutes)

Sometimes you may think your baby is waking up when they’re actually going through a phase of light sleep. They could be squirming, startling, fussing - or even crying - and still be asleep. Do not make the mistake of trying to comfort them during these moments, you’ll only awaken them further and delay them going back to sleep. Instead, if you let them fuss and even cry for a few minutes, they’ll learn to go back to sleep themselves without always relying on you.

With the goal of teaching good sleep habits, temporary crying is preferable over poor sleep habits that are far more harmful than a little crying.

Some babies cry 15min before falling asleep, others cry from 5min at one nap to an off-and-on 35min cry at another.

15min should be the cut off. If they cry longer than 15min, check on them. Pat them on the back & hold them for a moment before putting them back down.

Remember: You are not training your baby not to cry, but how to sleep!

Identifying Cry Patterns

Identifying & knowing your baby's cry patterns & disposition will help you discern real needs. Some babies have a nap time cry pattern like a bell curve: a gentle whimper building to a mild wail, which falls back to a whimper before then go to sleep. This cycle might last a total of 10-15min. Another pattern might be crying for 10min, then stopping, then starting again a minute or so later for another 5min before falling asleep. Another pattern might be a cry starting from a whimper, peaking at a full cry, and abruptly stopping & falling asleep.

Become a student of baby's cry patterns. When you do, you will know what is normal for them and you will know what is abnormal.

Cries to listen for:

Some crying is normal & expected, but you need to be alert for certain identifiable cries. Ex: a high-pitched, piercing cry may be a signal of either internal or external injury. If such a cry persists, consult your pediatrician.

A sudden change in cry pattern may be a warning of illness. Discuss with your pediatrician.

Cries for hunger or thirst are predictable with PDF babies.

A loud, piercing cry when waking in the middle of a nap may be caused by gas buildup or something in your breastmilk from something you ate. If this cry persists, physically check your baby & consult your pediatrician.

Responding to baby's cry

Normal cry cycles can last 15min, but abnormal cries should be responded to immediately.

With abnormal crying, follow these 3 steps:

1. Where is your Baby in their routine - is nap time finished, or is he in the middle of their nap needing to resettle? Do they need to go down for a nap? Have they been in the swing too long? Did they lose a toy? Did they spit up? Is it their fussy time of day? Determine first the cause & then respond appropriately
2. Listen for the type of cry - In the early days you will begin to recognize different tones & patterns in the crying. By listening you can determine the right response
3. Take Action - Take action, but remember sometimes the best action is no action at all (Ex: if baby is clean, fed & ready for nap, let them learn how to fall asleep alone, this may be exactly what they need. Do not get into a habit of nursing them to sleep! This is detrimental to establishing this healthy system). Take note of how long crying lasts.

Some Happy Baby Method mothers are surprised to learn seemingly endless bouts of crying only last a few minutes. There will be times when your PA (Parental Assessment) calls for picking up & holding baby, even if it is only to reassure them everything is ok. Sometimes there is no rhyme or reason behind baby's need for a hold.

When should I hold & comfort Baby?

Most holding & attention comes naturally, but parents should remember this basic question: What kind of comfort should I give my baby right now? A diaper change will comfort a wet baby. A feed will comfort a hungry baby. Holding will comfort a startled baby, & sleep will comfort a tired baby.

Chapter 7

Colic, Reflux & Inconsolable Babies

What happens when a baby does not follow the routine & shows fussiness beyond normal times? Maybe they cry for food but refuse the bottle. Maybe they cry in pain but reject your efforts to comfort. Maybe they spit up what looks like the entire meal at every feed. What should you do?

Here are 4 stories from our HBM community:

1. **ASHLEY**

- PROBLEM: "Ashley showed all the normal hunger signs but would nurse feverishly and suddenly stop. She would pull away & start screaming. I knew something was wrong, but what? We tried everything. I changed my diet, fed more often, fed less often, switched sides & burped often. Nothing helped. Sleep was not best, she slept 30min naps if i could get her to sleep at all. At night she would wake 4-5 times."
- SOLUTION: "Once Ashley was diagnosed with reflux, we knew what we were up against and that made things easier. Ashley improved greatly with the help of medication and by 6mo her acid reflux problem was gone. She then began to sleep through the night (within 3 days of training). Once she began sleeping through the night her napping routine improved. Now at 2 years old, she sleeps 12hrs/night and naps 2-3 hours/day."

2. **JOHN**

- PROBLEM: "John was spitting up large amounts after every feed from the first week. At 2 weeks old John was spitting up 40-50 times per day. There were times he would spit up so much I wondered if I should even try feeding him again fearing everything would just come right back up. He stayed on a 2hr feed routine for the first 3 months which completely destroyed his sleep cycles - and mine! I thought neither of us were ever going to get any rest."
- SOLUTION: "At his 3 month checkup, he was placed on Prevacid® in dissolvable pill form. This worked wonders. We finally were able to transition to crib sleeping and he began sleeping through the night. Finally at 15 months, he no longer needed the medication. At his 18-month checkup, he was in or able the 50% range for the first time ever."

3. **CYNTHIA**

- PROBLEM: "Cynthia would spit up 15-20min after each meal. At 3 weeks she had difficulty nursing and began crying during feeds. This was a traumatic event for us both. Although she slept fairly well, she would still wake up around 3am every night and struggled to put on weight."
- SOLUTION: "We took a list of symptoms to our pediatrician, who suspected reflux. She prescribed Zantac®. We saw a significant difference in just 2 days. As she began feeding better, night sleep also improved.

She continued nursing for 13 months. Once she started drinking from a cup, we stopped the medicine & the reflux was gone."

4. EDWARD

- PROBLEM: "Edward was born via c-section with healthy weight & condition. By the end of week 1, everything started downhill fast. He was very fussy & always seemed to be in pain and distressed. If I was lucky he would sleep for an hour and a half stretch, then wake up screaming covered in vomit. At his two-week checkup, he was weight & measured and we were told he was growing optimally. We relayed all of the problems he was facing to the doctor who told us it was just colic and a bit of reflux. When I tried insisting it was more, I was told there was nothing to worry about. Of course, everything wasn't fine. His condition got worse. We visited a gastroenterologist, who did an ultrasound of his abdomen and deduced Edward had a severe case of Gastroesophageal Reflux Disease (GERD)."

- SOLUTION: "Because of his healthy weight gain, our pediatrician chose medication over invasive procedures. The meds worked wonderfully. His reflux improved beautifully and his body began to relax. After a week on medication, he slept 12hrs through the night and has continued to do so since."

COLIC

Crying and Colic

There is a big difference between fussy babies and policy babies. Fussy babies have fussy times followed by relative peace and calm the rest of the day or night. Colicky babies seem irritable all the time, day and night. Symptoms of colic include piercing cries & signs of acute stomach distress - i.e. folding legs, flailing arms, inconsolable crying and passing gas. *Although symptoms may seem like a digestive disorder, it isn't.

Most research suggests that colic is the underdevelopment of the nervous system being unable to process the full range of stimuli among newborns at birth. This condition affects roughly 20% of infants. It shows up usually between weeks 2-4 & generally ends by month 3. While there are no significant medical issues related with real colic, it creates a lot of stress and anxiety in the home.

What can a Mother do?

As of yet there is no cure for colic, but all babies will outgrow it. Here are some suggestions to dealing with colic:

1. Consult your pediatrician and rule out any other potential medical causes for excessive crying or spitting up. Get a second opinion if your concerns are not being appropriately addressed.
2. All babies are different and respond to different measures. Find out what works for your baby and stay with it. Some mothers find giving a warm bath helps, or placing them in an infant swing. If bottle feeding, try

changing formula.

3. Breastfeeding moms may find certain foods in her diet trigger Baby's discomfort. Start by eliminating gas-producing foods (beans, broccoli, cauliflower, cabbage, onions, garlic, etc.) or spicy foods, dairy, caffeine and alcohol. Be systematic in your approach so you can single out specifically what is causing the issue. If food sensitivity is an issue, you will see noticeable difference in colic symptoms within a couple days. After a few weeks you can gradually reintroduce individual items back into your diet & monitor your Baby's reaction.
4. Avoid having your baby come in contact with secondhand smoke - especially with colic.
5. Pacifiers may bring comfort & help your baby relax. Some research suggests SIDS rates among infants who are given a pacifier are significantly lower.
6. Colicky babies need to be burped frequently. If bottle feeding, try a different bottle or nipple design to help reduce the amount of air your baby swallows during a feed. After each feed, lay your baby across your knees, stomach down & gently massage their back. This may relieve their discomfort and pressure
7. Blue light exposure may exacerbate colic symptoms & delay neurological development. Be sure to feed in a soothing environment .
8. Some babies are comforted by rhythmic motion and/or white noise. If so, prop them in a baby swing near continuous noise or vibration

Taking Care of You

First time parents find the early months extremely challenging, especially if they have a colicky baby. One of the best things you can do for your baby is take care of yourself. Keep your routine going, but involve trusted friends or family members to give you a break when feeling overwhelmed.

Remember this: your baby WILL outgrow colic

Reflux & GERD

One of the biggest medical risks associated with colic is that colic symptoms often mimic symptoms of more serious conditions like milk-protein allergies, lactose intolerance, Gastroesophageal Reflux (GER), and Gastroesophageal Reflux Disease (GERD).

GER causes asymptomatic spitting up and does not require medical treatment if the baby is growing properly

GERD causes intense pain and will lead to feeding aversion if not treated. GERD requires medical attention, usually in the form of medication, but sometimes requires surgery.

Both are highly manageable if treated correctly

Reflux

It is estimated 3-5% of newborns have mild to severe reflux symptoms for the first few months of life (Data collected from USA)

Reflux is usually due to an immature sphincter valve between the stomach and the esophagus. This valve allows us to swallow, burp, or vomit. An immature sphincter periodically relaxes, allowing stomach acid back up into the esophagus & throat, causing a burning sensation.

The condition can advance to where it causes weight loss or esophagitis. This is GERD.

Many babies with minor reflux are happy and thriving, they require little medical intervention.

They usually outgrow their symptoms without complications.

One of the most important indicators of GERD is the baby's inability to be consoled - crying because they are in extreme pain. Once medication is prescribed, you will see improvement within 2 days and a lot of improvement within 2 weeks (If symptoms persist, consult doctor immediately).

Colic, Reflux, and The Happy Baby Method

Many parents who are dealing with colic or reflux may assume this system will not work for them - but this isn't true!

The Happy Baby Method will help bring order to the chaotic situation. You will need to make minor adaptions to the routine to fit your unique situation, but the structure will be there to have your baby sleeping through the night as soon as possible.

Challenges in the Routine

1. Try to keep to 2.5-3hr FWS cycles.
2. A well-established sleep pattern will take longer to achieve with reflux, but it will come! All PDF-trained babies begin sleeping through the night, reflux or not, between 13-18 weeks.
3. Keep the baby's environment calm & quiet. Avoid bouncing, jiggling or excessive back patting

4. Don't worry if you aren't following the plan down to a T. You aren't competing with anyone! You are after the goal of achieving a full nighttime sleep, not the world record of fastest baby to get there.

Feed times & Wake times

1. Avoid two extremes: letting baby get too hungry & over-feeding them. Burp frequently!
2. Prop baby in an upright position after each feed for at least 30min, this will help with digestion.
3. If a feed is dragging out longer than 45min, stop the feed & give your baby some down time - possibly back to the crib. Don't worry if they fall asleep. Its better to wake them up early for the next feed than to go too long trying to achieve the full feed.
4. Some breastfeeding moms have an overflowing supply of milk. Their babies will adapt by swallowing faster and gulping, leading to excessive air swallowing. This exacerbates reflux. Recline in a lounge chair or lie down to allow gravity to slow the flow of milk. You can also use two fingers like scissors around your nipple to help regulate the flow.
5. Avoid overfeeding to reduce spitting up. With babies who spit up with reflux, the AAP suggests not offering another feed but simply waiting until the next one.
6. Bottle-fed babies who have reflux sometimes benefit from having formula thickened with rice cereal (check with your pediatrician first).
7. If you are recommended medicine by your pediatrician, check the side effects! Some medications induce stomach

cramps that appear to be colic.

8. Be sure to not pull the diaper too tight, this can put unnecessary pressure on them.

Sleeping

1. Try swaddling your baby, giving them a pacifier or changing their sleep position
2. If your baby is habitually waking up 45min into their nap screaming in pain, consider going in after 40min and gently rocking them through the cycle so your baby doesn't become over-stimulated by their crying.
3. For babies over 3months old, use the pacifier immediately upon waking. Sit, walk or rock them until they display signs of tiredness and try to put them back down.

Crying

1. Typical signs of reflux are crying through feeds, not latching on and very small feedings. Feed them immediately upon waking
2. If they are stressed during feeds, stop and relax them before continuing.
3. Reflux babies tend to be more comfortable in upright positions. AAP has observed the back position may increase crying.
4. One day at a time! Focus on the long-term goal of establishing your healthy FWS cycles. Some days will be great, others wont, but you have to focus on the long term goal.

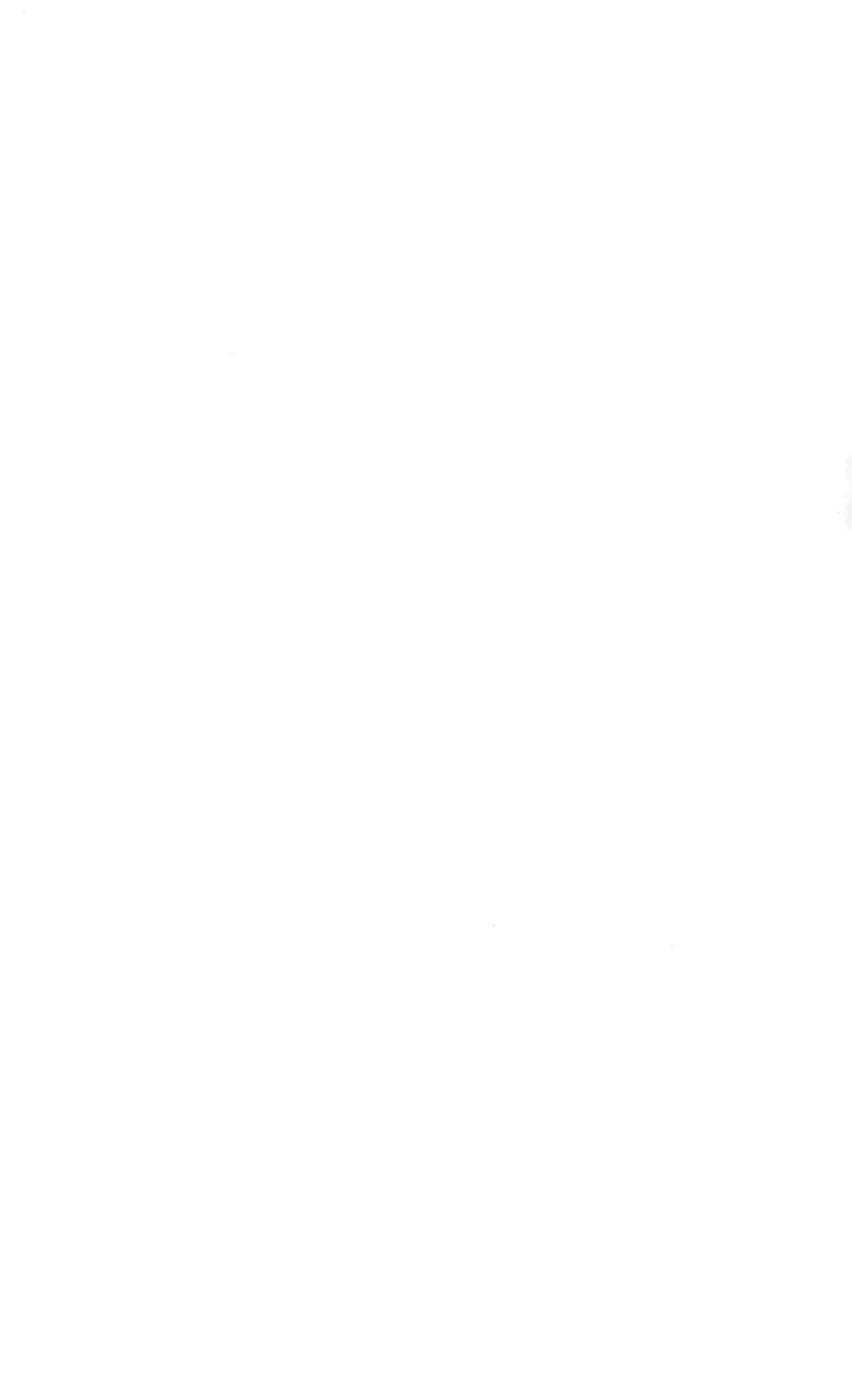

Lightning Source UK Ltd.
Milton Keynes UK
UKHW021839020720
365935UK00017B/359